GW00367852

miracle juices™

energize

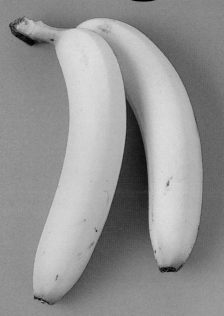

Safety Note

Energize should not be considered a replacement for
professional medical treatment; a physician should be
consulted on all matters relating to health. While the advice and
information in this book is believed to be accurate, the publisher
cannot accept any legal responsibility or liability for any injury
or illness sustained while following the advice in this book.

First published in Great Britain in 2002 by
Hamlyn, a division of Octopus Publishing Group Ltd
2–4 Heron Quays, London E14 4JP

Copyright © Octopus Publishing Group Ltd 2002

ISBN 0 600 60695 3

A CIP catalogue record for this book is available
from the British Library

Printed and bound in China

10 9 8 7 6 5 4 3 2 1

Contents

introduction

Are you always full of energy, bursting to get out there and enjoy every moment life has to offer, or do you often find yourself complaining that you are tired, feeling irritable and lacking enthusiasm? If it is the latter, the answer could lie in the type of food you are eating, because food provides our major source of energy. In order to move, breathe and maintain brain power, we need to consume the right foodstuffs, and many of us undermine this valuable fuel by eating junk food and skipping meals. Add to this a high consumption of alcohol, tea and coffee, sugary drinks, chocolate and smoking and you will be severely limiting your ability to perform at your peak, particularly in times of stress when energy requirements are greater than usual.

Where does our energy come from?

Food is converted into energy during the process of digestion. It is broken down into glucose which is carried to the liver, where it is filtered and stored as glycogen. The pituitary gland in the brain stimulates hormonal releases from the adrenal glands and pancreas, which cause the liver to release the glucose back into the bloodstream when it is needed and it is delivered to whichever organs and muscles require it.

The process of keeping our organs and muscles supplied with the fuel they need is known as blood sugar management. Many different nutrients are required for energy production and a variety of different foods provide the essential blend. Carbohydrates are the key as they are most easily converted into glucose; proteins and fats provide a secondary source of energy, but are equally vital as they provide essential nutrients.

Getting the balance right

The balance between carbohydrates and protein is the lynchpin for sustainable energy and the optimal balance for each person depends on their lifestyle. If you are inactive, elderly or recuperating from an illness, your ratio of protein to carbohydrate should be 1:2. If you lead an active life, then your ideal ratio would be 1:1. Energy requirements are also higher during pregnancy, childhood, puberty and during periods of stress.

glycaemic index

All foods have what is known as a glycaemic index, or GI. This indicates the speed with which they release their sugars into the body. The higher the GI, the quicker the impact on blood sugar levels. Refined foods such as white bread, white rice, sweets and chocolate, commercial cereals and canned drinks all have a high glycaemic value. They will provide an immediate sugar surge, but deplete the body's energy reserves very quickly, leaving a person with less energy than before. It is better to eat foods with a low to moderate GI which supply a constant release of sugar throughout the day.

Low GI foods
- Whole grains (rye, quinoa, millet)
- Soya beans, haricot beans, butter beans, kidney beans
- Chickpeas, lentils
- Yogurt
- Apples, pears, oranges, kiwifruit, bananas
- Oats
- Wholemeal pasta
- Raw root vegetables

Medium GI foods
- Popcorn
- Sweetcorn
- Potatoes
- Mangoes, apricots, papaya
- Muesli
- Brown rice
- Raisins
- Corn chips

Symptoms of energy imbalance

- Depression
- Irritability
- Mood swings
- Premenstrual tension
- Angry outbursts
- Anxiety and nervousness
- Fatigue
- Lack of concentration
- Continual thirst
- Constant craving for sugar, bread or carbohydrates throughout the day
- Feelings of sluggishness and heaviness in the mornings
- High consumption of stimulants such as tea, coffee, alcohol and carbonated drinks

Boosting energy

Juicing raw vegetables and fruit is a great way to boost energy. Because juices contain no fibre to slow down digestion, the nutrients are readily absorbed and the release of glucose into the bloodstream is rapid. But, to avoid energy peaks and troughs, don't forget to nibble on healthy snacks to help balance blood sugar throughout the day and sustain that vital energy.

The following are good examples.

- Nuts and dried fruit
- Low-fat yogurt with pumpkin seeds and wheatgerm
- Oat and wheatgerm flapjacks
- Crispbread or oatcakes with cheese
- Avocado dip with rice cakes
- Raw vegetables with yogurt or soured cream
- Apple
- Hummus and raw carrot

key nutrients

Nutrient	Function	Sources	Recommended Daily Dosage
Vitamin B1 (thiamine)	Helps convert carbohydrates to glucose; ensures proper oxygenation of the blood for optimal energy release	Brewer's yeast, rice bran, whole grains, raw wheatgerm, green and yellow vegetables, fruit, milk	1.2–1.4 mg (this can be raised to 10–50 mg per day to increase wellbeing)
Vitamin B3 (niacin)	Aids in the metabolism of macronutrients; strengthens digestion; improves blood circulation	Liver, brewer's yeast, raw wheatgerm, fish, eggs, peanuts, dried fruits, avocados	13–18 mg
Vitamin B5 (pantothenic acid)	Stimulates adrenal function; prevents fatigue; reduces stress	Cod roe, meat, raw wheatgerm, whole grains, beans, molasses, nuts, brewer's yeast	10 mg (increase to 30–50 mg when energy is low)
Vitamin B6 (pyridoxine)	Necessary for release of glycogen from the liver when muscles need energy	Brewer's yeast, raw wheatgerm, liver, molasses, cabbage, milk, eggs	1.8–2.2 mg (some nutritionists recommend up to 25 mg)
Vitamin B12 (pyridoxine)	Increases energy; improves brain function; maintains a healthy nervous system	Liver and kidney, meat, eggs, dairy products, spirulina	3 mcg

Nutrient	Function	Sources	Recommended Daily Dosage
Folic acid	Necessary for brain function; works as a coenzyme in the breakdown and utilization of proteins	Green leafy vegetables, liver, egg yolk, carrots, cantaloupe melon, pumpkin, avocados, beans	400 mcg
Vitamin C (ascorbic acid)	Helps to alleviate fatigue, anxiety and depression by assisting in the formation of norepinephrine; used up rapidly by the body during periods of stress	Citrus fruits, peppers, broccoli, tomatoes, cabbage, green leafy vegetables, melons, yams, potatoes	60 mg (many nutritionists recommend 1000–2000 mg to promote immunity, general health and boost energy levels)
Magnesium	Helps to balance blood sugar levels and reduce cravings for stimulants; very effective muscle relaxant; vital for energy production of glucose; helps utilize B complex and C vitamins in the body	Figs, lemons, grapefruits, sweetcorn, nuts, apples, raw wheatgerm, green vegetables	350 mg
Zinc	Involved in carbohydrate metabolism; absorption and action of the B complex vitamins; helps energy production	Raw oysters, meat, fish, raw wheatgerm, mushrooms, pumpkin seeds, egg yolks, dried legumes, milk	15 mg

why juice?

Vital vitamins and minerals such as antioxidants, vitamins A, B, C and E, folic acid, potassium, calcium, magnesium, zinc and amino acids are present in fresh fruits and vegetables, and are all necessary for optimum health. Because juicing removes the indigestible fibre in fruits and vegetables, the nutrients are available to the body in much larger quantities than if the piece of fruit or vegetable were eaten whole. For example, when you eat a raw carrot you are able to assimilate only about 1 per cent of the available beta-carotene, because many of the nutrients are trapped in the fibre. When a carrot is juiced, thereby removing the fibre, nearly 100 per cent of the beta-carotene can be assimilated. Juicing several types of fruits and vegetables on a daily basis is therefore an easy way to ensure that your body receives its full quota of these vital vitamins and minerals.

In addition, fruits and vegetables provide another substance absolutely essential for good health — water. Most people don't consume enough water. In fact, many of the fluids we drink — coffee, tea, soft drinks, alcoholic beverages and artificially flavoured drinks — contain substances that require extra water for the body to eliminate, and tend to be dehydrating. Fruit and vegetable juices are free of these unnecessary substances.

Your health

A diet high in fruits and vegetables can prevent and help to cure a wide range of ailments. At the cutting edge of nutritional research are the plant chemicals known as phytochemicals, which hold the key to preventing deadly diseases such as cancer and heart disease, and others such as asthma, arthritis and allergies.

Although juicing benefits your overall health and wellbeing, it should be used only to complement your daily eating plan. You must still eat enough from the other food groups (such as grains, dairy food and pulses) to ensure your body maintains strong bones and healthy cells. If you are following a specially prescribed diet, or are under medical supervision, it is essential that you discuss any drastic changes with your health practitioner before beginning any type of new health regime.

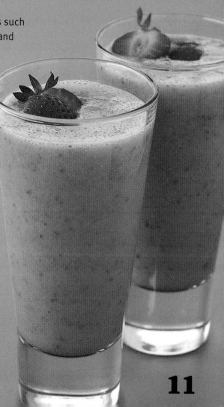

how to juice

Available in a variety of models, juicers work by separating the fruit and vegetable juice from the pulp. Choose a juicer with a reputable brand name, that has an opening big enough for larger fruits and vegetables, and make sure it is easy to take apart and clean, otherwise you may become discouraged from using it.

Types of juicer

A citrus juicer or lemon squeezer is ideal for extracting the juice from oranges, lemons, limes and grapefruit. Pure citrus juice has a high acid content and is best used diluted.

Centrifugal juicers are the most widely used and affordable juicers available. Fresh fruits and vegetables are fed into a rapidly spinning grater, and the pulp separated from the juice by centrifugal force. The pulp is retained in the machine while the juice runs into a separate jug. A centrifugal juicer produces less juice than the more expensive masticating juicer, which works by pulverizing fruits and vegetables, and pushing them through a wire mesh with immense force.

To make smoothies you will need a blender or food processor, as instructed in some recipes.

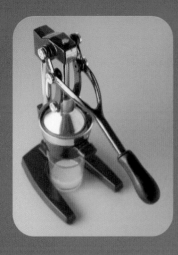

to two parts water will lessen any staining produced by the fruits and vegetables.

Preparing produce for juicing

It is best to prepare ingredients just before juicing so that fewer nutrients are lost through oxidization. Cut or tear foods into manageable pieces for juicing. If the ingredients are not organic, do not include stems, skins or roots, but if the produce is organic, you can put everything in the juicer. However, don't include the skins from pineapple, mango, papaya, citrus fruit and banana, and remove the stones from avocados, apricots, peaches, mangoes and plums. You can include melon seeds, particularly watermelon, as these are full of juice. For grape juice, choose green grapes with an amber tinge or black grapes with a darkish bloom. Leave the pith on lemons for the pectin content.

Cleaning the juicer

Clean your juicing machine thoroughly, as any residue left may harbour bacterial growth — a toothbrush or nailbrush works well for removing stubborn residual pulp. Leaving the equipment to soak in warm soapy water will loosen the residue from those hard-to-reach places. A solution made up of one part white vinegar

13

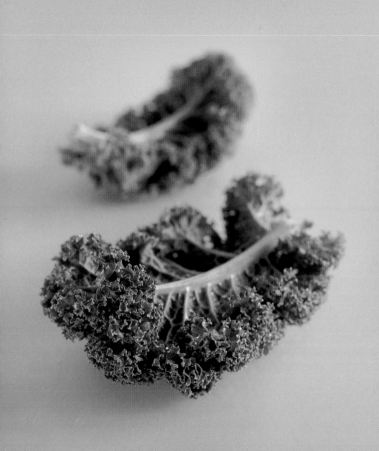

invigorate

Carrots, beetroots and oranges are all high in vitamins A and C, antioxidants and phytonutrients. This juice is also a rich source of potassium. A real tonic which should give your energy levels a boost.

power pack

250 g (8 oz) carrot
125 g (4 oz) beetroot
1 orange
125 g (4 oz) strawberries

Juice the carrot, beetroot and orange. Put the juice into a blender with a couple of ice cubes and the strawberries. Whizz for 20 seconds and serve in a tall glass. Decorate with strips of orange rind, if liked.
Makes 200 ml (7 fl oz)

Nutritional values

- Kcals 244
- Carbohydrate 55 g
- Protein 7 g
- Vitamin C 230 mg
- Vitamin A 2040 IU
- Magnesium 55 mg
- Zinc 1 mg

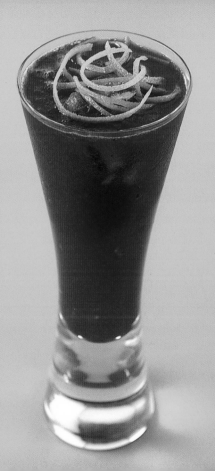

17

Spirulina is one the best sources of vitamin B12, which is essential for the functioning of all cells. Wheatgrass is high in chlorophyll, which combats anaemia. Kale has as much usable calcium as milk. This juice is a great energy booster with nutritional benefits that far outweigh its flavour.

kale and hearty

25 g (1 oz) kale
100 g (3½ oz) wheatgrass
1 teaspoon spirulina

Juice the kale and the wheatgrass, and stir in the spirulina powder. Serve in a small glass decorated with wheatgrass blades.
Makes 50 ml (2 fl oz)

Nutritional values

- Kcals 48
- Carbohydrate 25 g
- Protein 7 g
- Vitamin C 114 mg
- Vitamin A 1186 IU
- Magnesium 64 mg
- Zinc 2 mg

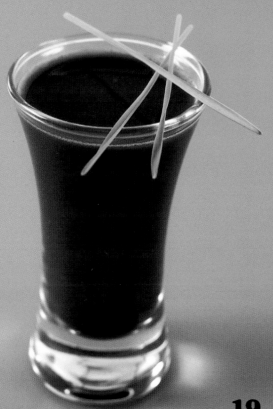

19

High in carbohydrate, this juice is a great energy giver, so it is most suitable after exercise. It can also be a good choice before exercise, however, when high levels of energy will be required. It is also an excellent source of vitamins A and C, potassium, magnesium and phosphorus, and provides useful amounts of iron. To counteract the sweetness of the mango it's best to use a tart variety of apple, such as a Worcester.

energy bubble

3 apples, preferably red
1 mango
2 passion fruit

Wash the apples, peel the mango and remove the stone. Slice the passion fruit in half, scoop out the flesh and discard the seeds. Juice all the ingredients. Pour the juice into a glass and add some ice cubes. Decorate with apple slices, if liked.

Makes 300 ml (½ pint)

Nutritional values

- Kcals 237
- Carbohydrate 58 g
- Protein 3 g
- Vitamin C 80 mg
- Vitamin A 298 IU
- Magnesium 43 mg
- Zinc 1 mg

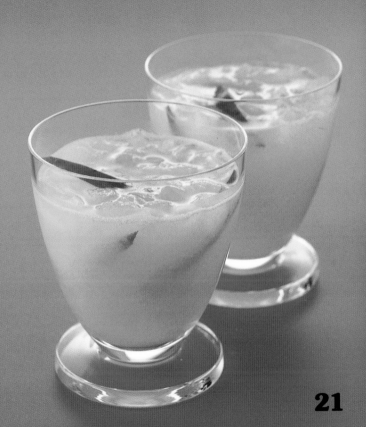

21

This juice contains cinnamon, which is renowned for stabilizing blood sugar.
To add a boost of glucose-regulating chromium, stir 1 tablespoon of raw wheatgerm
into the finished juice. This juice can help cure hypoglycaemia or very low blood
sugar levels which can cause fatigue, light-headedness and depression.

energy
burst

125 g (4 oz) spinach
250 g (8 oz) apple
100 g (3½ oz) yellow
  pepper
pinch of cinnamon

Juice the spinach, apple and pepper, then stir in the cinnamon. Serve in a glass and add a cinnamon stick for decoration, if liked.

Makes 200 ml (7 fl oz)

Nutritional values

- Kcals 175
- Carbohydrate 375 g
- Protein 6 g
- Vitamin C 178 mg
- Vitamin A 466 IU
- Magnesium 98 mg
- Zinc 1 mg

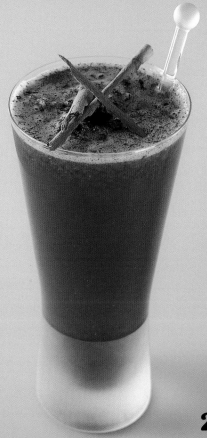

23

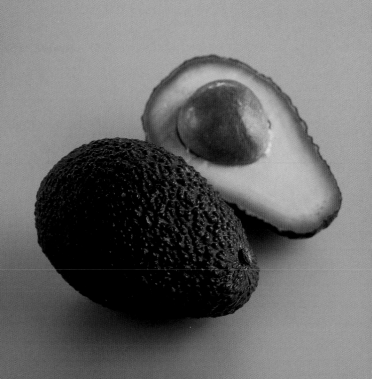

get up and go

We would run out of paper listing the nutritional aspects of this juice.
Basically it is a great all-round energy booster and the perfect way to perk up your senses, day or night.

magnificent 7

90 g (3 oz) carrot
50 g (2 oz) green pepper
25 g (1 oz) spinach
25 g (1 oz) onion
50 g (2 oz) celery
90 g (3 oz) cucumber
50 g (2 oz) tomato
sea salt and pepper

Juice all the ingredients and season with sea salt and pepper. If liked, decorate with tomato quarters.
Makes 200 ml (7 fl oz)

Nutritional values

- Kcals 75
- Carbohydrate 14 g
- Protein 3 g
- Vitamin C 87 mg
- Vitamin A 872 IU
- Magnesium 35 mg
- Zinc 1 mg

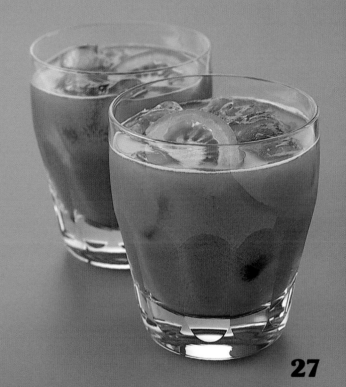

A good drink to choose before or after most activities including high-energy sports. Pineapples contain an enzyme, bromelain, that breaks down protein. This juice is rich in B vitamins which help to release energy from carbohydrate. It is an excellent source of vitamins C, B1 and B6, calcium and copper.

sky high

2 pears
½ lime
¼ pineapple, about
215 g (7½ oz)
peeled flesh

Juice all the fruit, pour into a glass and add some ice cubes, if wished. Decorate with pieces of pineapple, if liked.
Makes 300 ml (½ pint)

Nutritional values

- Kcals 211
- Carbohydrate 53 g
- Protein 2 g
- Vitamin C 55 mg
- Vitamin A 10 IU
- Magnesium 57 mg
- Zinc 1 mg

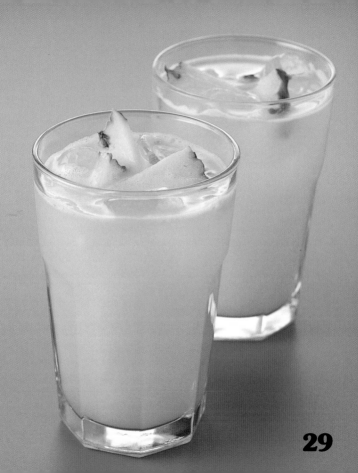

29

High in potassium, vitamin C, vitamin B12 and essential fatty acids, this is a thick shake with a punch. Basically, it is nutritious food, fast. These fruits, in particular the banana, create a feeling of fullness as well as helping to rebalance your sugar levels and thus your energy levels. Your sugar levels will also be helped by the protein in the linseeds. The high levels of vitamin B in the juice will also increase your energy.

high kick

250 g (8 oz) strawberries
125 g (4 oz) kiwifruit
100 g (3½ oz) banana
1 tablespoon spirulina
1 tablespoon linseeds

Juice the strawberries and kiwifruit and whizz in a blender with the banana, spirulina, linseeds and a couple of ice cubes. Decorate with redcurrants, if liked.

Makes 200 ml (7 fl oz)

Nutritional values

- Kcals 300
- Carbohydrate 54 g
- Protein 15 g
- Vitamin C 277 mg
- Vitamin A 1503 IU
- Magnesium 132 mg
- Zinc 1 mg

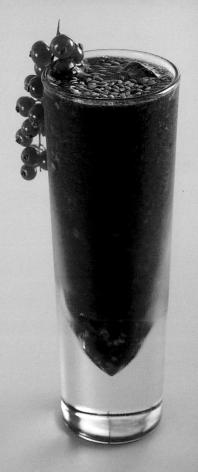

31

This juice provides good amounts of calcium and iron, which make it an excellent energy booster before or during most types of exercise, or just when you need a boost. Calcium is important for good bone health, while the iron helps to prevent fatigue. It is an excellent source of vitamins C, B1 and B2, niacin, B6, folic acid, copper, potassium, calcium, magnesium and phosphorus.

berry bouncer

100 g (3½ oz) strawberries
75 g (3 oz) redcurrants
½ orange
125 ml (4 fl oz) water
½ teaspoon clear honey (optional)

Hull the strawberries and redcurrants, and peel the orange. Juice the fruit, then add the water. Pour into a glass, stir in the honey, if using, and add some ice cubes. Decorate with redcurrants, if liked.

Makes 250 ml (8 fl oz)

Nutritional values

- Kcals 65
- Carbohydrate 14 g
- Protein 2 g
- Vitamin C 139 mg
- Vitamin A 4 IU
- Magnesium 26 mg
- Zinc 1 mg

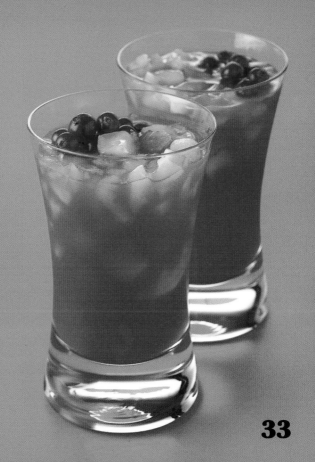

33

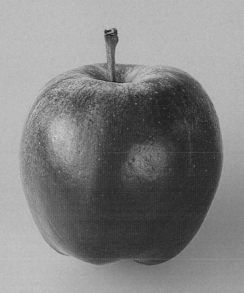

activate

High in water, melons add a refreshing flavour to juices. This juice has quite a high carbohydrate content, so it is good for providing fuel for sports activities. It is an excellent source of vitamins C, B1, B2 and B6, copper, potassium, magnesium and phosphorus and provides useful amounts of calcium. Melon and pineapple are both quite sweet so it's best to use a tart variety of apple such as Granny Smith or Worcester.

liven up

**½ Galia melon, about
    400 g (13 oz)**
**¼ pineapple, about 215 g
    (7½ oz) peeled flesh**
1 apple

Remove the skin and seeds from the melon. Juice all the ingredients, pour into a glass and add a couple of ice cubes. Decorate with apple slices, if liked.
Makes 300 ml (½ pint)

Nutritional values

- Kcals 216
- Carbohydrate 52 g
- Protein 3 g
- Vitamin C 90 mg
- Vitamin A 5 IU
- Magnesium 86 mg
- Zinc 1 mg

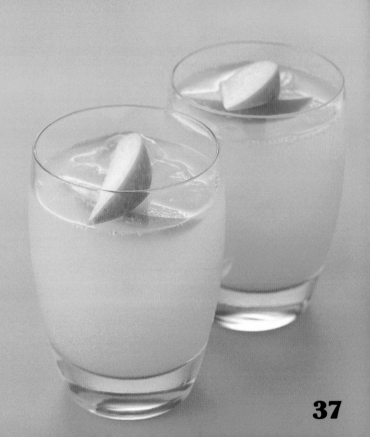

This high-carbohydrate, low-fat smoothie is a great choice for refuelling and soothing tired muscles. Bananas are high in potassium, a vital mineral for muscle and nerve function, which also helps to regulate blood pressure. It is also an excellent source of vitamins C, B1 and B6, folic acid, magnesium and phosphorus.

all nighter

1 small ripe banana
75 g (3 oz) strawberries
250 ml (8 fl oz) orange
   juice

Peel the banana and strawberries. Put the fruit into a freezer container and freeze for at least 2 hours or overnight. Place the frozen fruit and the orange juice in a food processor or blender and process until thick. Decorate with strawberries, if liked, and serve immediately.

Makes 400 ml (14 fl oz)

Nutritional values

- Kcals 180
- Carbohydrate 43 g
- Protein 3 g
- Vitamin C 187 mg
- Vitamin A 7 IU
- Magnesium 65 mg
- Zinc 0.5 mg

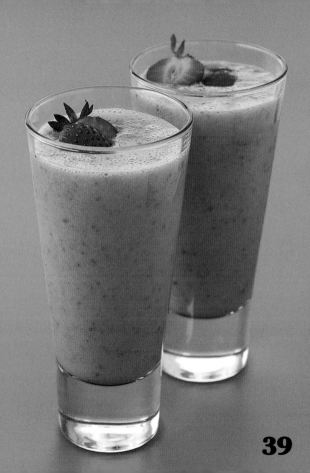

This juice contains large amounts of carbohydrate, essential for refuelling energy stores. The addition of honey gives an extra energy boost. It is an excellent source of vitamins C, B1, B2 and B6, folic acid, calcium, copper and potassium, magnesium and phosphorus.

live wire

2 oranges
1 red apple
1 pear
1 teaspoon clear honey (optional)

Peel the oranges, juice the flesh with the apple and pear and pour the juice into a glass. Stir in the honey, if using, and add a couple of ice cubes. Decorate with thin orange slices, if liked.

Makes 350 ml (12 fl oz)

Nutritional values

- Kcals 225
- Carbohydrate 54 g
- Protein 4 g
- Vitamin C 188 mg
- Vitamin A 13 IU
- Magnesium 48 mg
- Zinc 1 mg

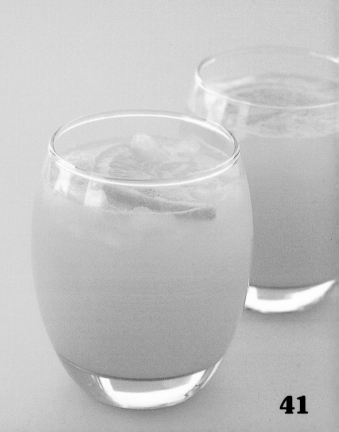

Kiwifruit are an excellent source of vitamin C. This juice will help get you through the day as it contains large amounts of carbohydrate for energy release, plus a hefty amount of vitamin C which may help to increase oxygen uptake and energy production. It is also a good source of vitamins B1 and B6, copper, potassium, magnesium and phosphorus and also provides useful amounts of calcium.

battery charge

2 kiwifruit
300 g (10 oz) seedless
**   green grapes**

Peel the kiwifruit and juice them with the grapes. Pour the juice into a glass and add a couple of ice cubes. Decorate with kiwifruit slices, if liked.
Makes 300 ml (½ pint)

Nutritional values

- Kcals 239
- Carbohydrate 59 g
- Protein 3 g
- Vitamin C 80 mg
- Vitamin A 10 IU
- Magnesium 39 mg
- Zinc 1 mg

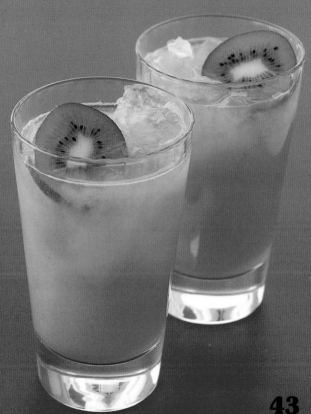

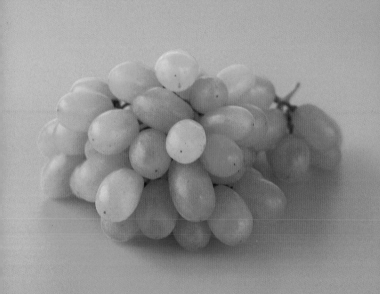

kick start

This isotonic juice is particularly suitable during exercise when a thirst-quenching drink is required. Grapes are a good source of potassium and make the perfect energy snack. This juice is an excellent source of vitamins C, B1 and B6, copper, magnesium and phosphorus.

marathon man

¼ Galia melon, about 150 g (5 oz)
75 g (3 oz) seedless green grapes
150 ml (¼ pint) water

Remove the skin and seeds from the melon and juice the fruit. Add the water, pour the juice into a glass and add some ice cubes. Decorate with sliced grapes, if liked.

Makes 300 ml (½ pint)

Nutritional values

- Kcals 87
- Carbohydrate 22 g
- Protein 1 g
- Vitamin C 25 mg
- Vitamin A 1 IU
- Magnesium 24 mg
- Zinc 0.5 mg

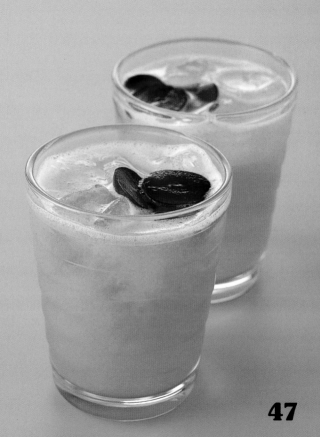

Bananas provide carbohydrate and energy, while avocados supply the body with healthy unsaturated fats. Just one avocado also provides around half the recommended daily intake of vitamin B6. This smoothie is an excellent source of vitamins C, E, B1, B2, B6 and B12, as well as folic acid, calcium, potassium, copper, zinc, magnesium and phosphorus. Drinking this will help to fuel the body and maintain good energy levels. Using skimmed milk helps keep down the overall fat content.

round the clock

1 small ripe avocado
1 small ripe banana
250 ml (8 fl oz) skimmed milk

Peel and stone the avocado, and peel the banana. Place the avocado, banana and milk in a food processor or blender and process until smooth. Pour into a glass, add a couple of ice cubes and drink immediately.
Makes 400 ml (14 fl oz)

Nutritional values

- Kcals 349
- Carbohydrate 33 g
- Protein 11 g
- Vitamin C 17 mg
- Vitamin A 5 IU
- Magnesium 80 mg
- Zinc 2 mg

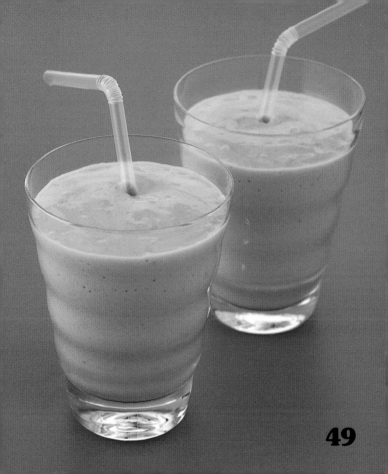

This smoothie is a good choice after exercise, when you need a boost. It will help refuel glycogen stores in the muscles and is rich in B vitamins, which help the body to optimize energy production and performance. It is also an excellent source of vitamins A, B1, B2, B6 and C, copper, potassium, magnesium and phosphorus, and provides useful amounts of iron.

rocket fuel

1 ripe mango
300 ml (½ pint) pineapple juice
rind and juice of ½ lime

Peel and stone the mango, roughly chop the flesh and put it in a freezer container. Freeze for at least 2 hours or overnight. Place the frozen mango in a food processor or blender with the pineapple juice and lime rind and juice and process until thick. Decorate with lime wedges, if liked, and serve immediately.

Nutritional values

Makes 400 ml (14 fl oz)

- Kcals 213
- Carbohydrate 54 g
- Protein 2 g
- Vitamin C 108 mg
- Vitamin A 273 IU
- Magnesium 41 mg
- Zinc 1 mg

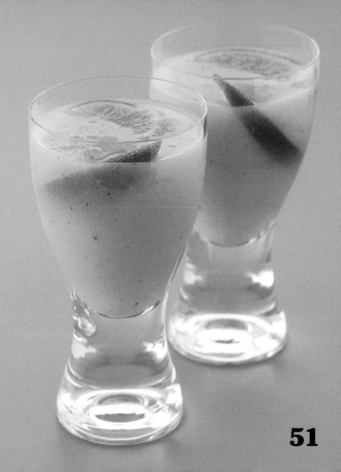

51

The combination of bananas, ground almonds and soya milk makes this a highly nutritious drink. It is best to use very ripe bananas (very yellow skin with black spots) as less ripe ones are largely indigestible. Almonds are an excellent source of vitamin E as well as the minerals calcium, magnesium, phosphorus and copper. They also help to increase the protein content of this drink, which is an excellent source of vitamins C, E, B1, B2 and B6, niacin, folic acid, copper, potassium, zinc, magnesium, phosphorus and provides useful amounts of calcium.

jumping jack

1 very ripe banana
250 ml (8 fl oz) soya milk
20 g (¾ oz) ground almonds
pinch of ground cinnamon
a little honey (optional)

Peel and slice the banana, put it into a freezer container and freeze for at least 2 hours or overnight. Place the frozen banana, soya milk, ground almonds and cinnamon in a food processor or blender, add the honey, if using, and process until thick and frothy. Pour into a glass and serve immediately with ice cubes and decorate with ground cinnamon.
Makes 300 ml (½ pint)

Nutritional values

- Kcals 315
- Carbohydrate 47 g
- Protein 9 g
- Vitamin C 11 mg
- Vitamin A 2 IU
- Magnesium 110 mg
- Zinc 1 mg

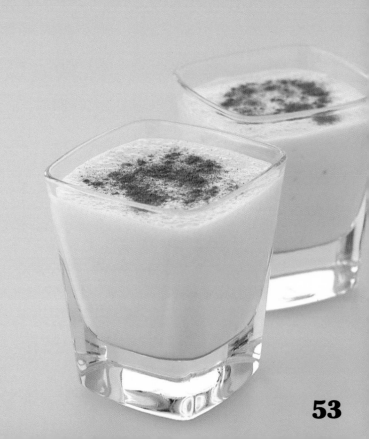

53

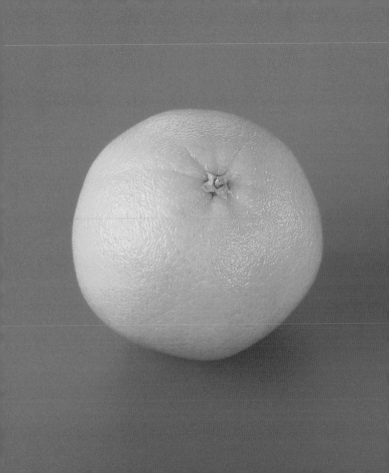

revitalize

Dried apricots have a good concentration of beta-carotene, potassium and iron, making them useful for refuelling muscles and boosting energy levels. Many brands of dried apricots are preserved using sulphur dioxide, which can trigger asthma attacks. To avoid this, check the packaging before you buy, or rinse the apricots well before eating them. This smoothie is an excellent source of vitamins C, B1 and B6, copper, potassium, magnesium and phosphorus and provides useful amounts of calcium and iron.

big boost

65 g (2½ oz) ready-to-eat dried apricots
350 ml (12 fl oz) pineapple juice

Roughly chop the apricots and put them in a large bowl. Pour the pineapple juice over them, cover the bowl and allow to stand overnight. Tip the contents of the bowl into a food processor or blender and process until smooth. Add a couple of ice cubes and drink immediately.

Makes 350 ml (12 fl oz)

Nutritional values

- Kcals 246
- Carbohydrate 61 g
- Protein 4 g
- Vitamin C 39 mg
- Vitamin A 38 IU
- Magnesium 49 mg
- Zinc 1 mg

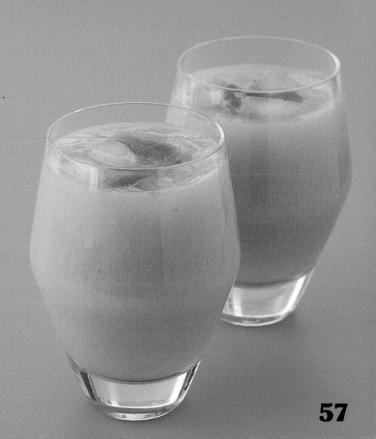

Containing high levels of carbohydrate for energy, and calcium for bone health and strength, this smoothie is ideal for people who do a lot of exercise. Cranberry juice is also a natural way to fight urinary tract infections. This smoothie is an excellent source of vitamins A, C, B1, B2, B6 and B12, folic acid, calcium, zinc, potassium, magnesium and phosphorus and also provides useful amounts of iron.

high flyer

1 ripe mango
200 ml (7 fl oz) cranberry juice
150 g (5 oz) peach yogurt

Peel and stone the mango and place the flesh in a food processor or blender with the cranberry juice and yogurt and process until smooth. Pour into a glass, add some ice cubes, decorate with cranberries, if liked, and drink immediately.
Makes 400 ml (14 fl oz)

Nutritional values

- Kcals 319
- Carbohydrate 70 g
- Protein 7 g
- Vitamin C 117 mg
- Vitamin A 280 IU
- Magnesium 42 mg
- Zinc 1 mg

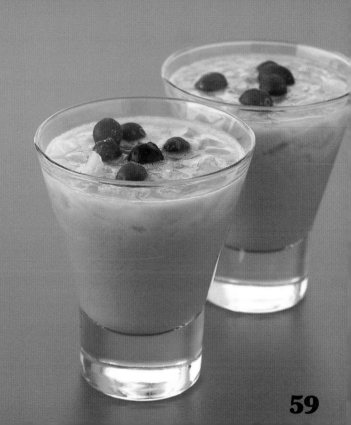

As it contains useful amounts of calcium, iron and carbohydrate and has low fat levels, this smoothie replaces energy and raises iron levels, while also helping to maintain bone health. It is an excellent source of vitamins A, C, B1, B2 and B6, folic acid, copper, potassium, magnesium and phosphorus.

quick hit

125 g (4 oz) strawberries
1 small ripe mango
300 ml (½ pint) orange
   juice

Hull the strawberries, place them in a freezer container and freeze for 2 hours or overnight. Peel and stone the mango, roughly chop the flesh and place it in a food processor or blender with the strawberries and orange juice and process until thick. Decorate with slices of mango, if liked, and serve immediately.
Makes 400 ml (14 fl oz)

Nutritional values

- Kcals 213
- Carbohydrate 52 g
- Protein 4 g
- Vitamin C 290 mg
- Vitamin A 258 IU
- Magnesium 67 mg
- Zinc 0.5 mg

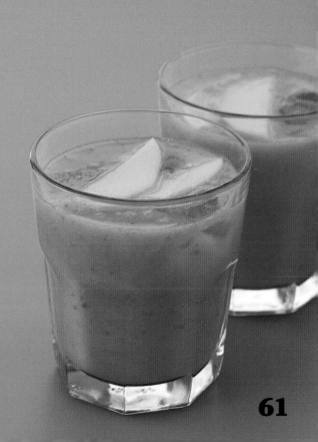

Versatility is the key to this smoothie. It is likely to be well absorbed as it is isotonic, and provides a good energy boost. Adding yogurt to a smoothie is an effective way to increase its content of calcium, which is essential for bone health and strength. Bananas and mangoes supply fibre, making this a filling and satisfying smoothie. It is an excellent source of vitamins A, C, B1, B2 and B6, folic acid, potassium, copper, magnesium and phosphorus.

bionic tonic

1 small banana
½ large ripe mango
75 g (3 oz) natural bio yogurt
150 ml (¼ pint) pineapple juice

Peel and slice the banana then put it in a freezer container and freeze for at least 2 hours or overnight. Peel and stone the mango, roughly chop the flesh and place it in a food processor or blender with the frozen banana, yogurt and pineapple juice. Process until smooth and serve immediately, decorated with pineapple chunks, if liked.

Makes 300 ml (½ pint)

Nutritional values

- Kcals 240
- Carbohydrate 50 g
- Protein 6 g
- Vitamin C 56 mg
- Vitamin A 161 IU
- Magnesium 60 mg
- Zinc 1 mg

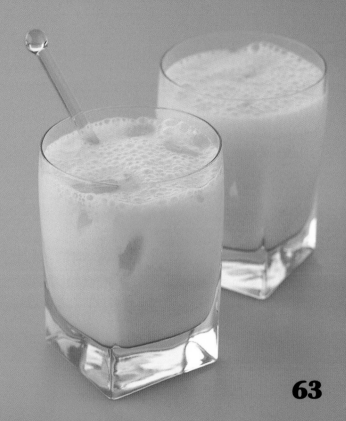

63

index

acknowledgements

The publisher would like to thank The Juicer Company
for the loan of The Champion juicer and the Orange X
citrus juicer (featured on pages 12 and 13).

The Juicer Company
28 Shambles
York
YO1 7LX
Tel: (01904) 541541
www.thejuicercompany.co.uk

Executive Editor Nicola Hill
Editor Abi Rowsell
Executive Art Editor Geoff Fennell
Designer Sue Michniewicz
Senior Production Controller Jo Sim
Photographer Stephen Conroy
Home Economist David Morgan
Stylist Angela Swaffield
All photographs © Octopus
Publishing Group Ltd